Dr. Sebi Recipes

For Everyone

A Complete Guide With Dr. Sebi's Recipes That Will Boost your Immune System and Change your Life Forever

Daphne Mitchell

Disclaimer Notice:

Please note the information contained within this document is for educational and entertainment purposes only. All effort has been executed to present accurate, up to date, and reliable, complete information. No warranties of any kind are declared or implied. Readers acknowledge that the author is not engaging in the rendering of legal, financial, medical or professional advice. The content within this book has been derived from various sources. Please consult a licensed professional before attempting any techniques outlined in this book.

By reading this document, the reader agrees that under no circumstances is the author responsible for any losses, direct or indirect, which are incurred as a result of the use of information contained within this document, including, but not limited to, errors, omissions, or inaccuracies.

Table of Content

Introduction

Thank You For Purchasing **Dr. Sebi Diet Cookbook: The Essential Step-By-Step Guide to the Alkaline Diet, Including a Simple Recipes Based on Vegetables, Herbs, and Soy**

A famous plant-based diet plan was formulated by the late Dr. Sebi, known by his name the Sebi diet, also known as the Sebi alkaline diet. This diet helps remove toxic waste in the body by alkalizing the blood. It is believed that this process revitalizes the cells. The diet normally depends, along with several supplements, on the consumption of a limited list of approved foods. Dr. Sebi argued that for more than 400 years, Western medical science has been treating diseases incorrectly, with very rare cures. Sebi argued that diseases are caused by host infection due to chemical treatment practices because this technique has been adopted inherently flawed in society. As a more effective and intuitive approach, Dr. Sebi refutes this technique by referring to the African philosophy, normally called African Bio-mineral Balance. The method promoted by Sebi suggests that if a mucous membrane is damaged, disease is induced in the body. When this happens, a drastic accumulation of this mucus is produced, which in turn creates disease. So, what is Sebi's answer or what is the alternative way to deal with this problem?

Prevention of these problems of mucus accumulation in the body depends on diet. The famous African Bio-mineral Balance philosophy assumes that disease can only occur in an acidic cli-mate. Dr. Sebi's recommended remedy is to de-develop a diet plan that focuses primarily on developing an alka-line deficiency. Like many other modern diets, plants are more focused with alkaline; because plants are natu-rally alkaline.

Dr. Sebi states that the alkaline diet develops an atmosphere in which infections cannot flourish. He also claims that African Bio-mineral-Balance rejuvenates damaged cellular tissue in the body. Dr. Sebi has developed a detoxifying cleansing process that purifies every cell in the body. The expectation is that the human body will begin the process of cellular rejuvenation. Her al-kaline diet, which is primarily based on the famous African Bio-Mineral theory was developed by Alfredo Darrington Bowman, also a self-taught herbalist better known as Dr. Sebi. Although Sebi was not properly a medical doctor and did not possess any doctoral degree. Without depending on standard Western medicine, Sebi built this diet for anyone who wishes to naturally cure or prevent disease and improve health.

According to Dr. Sebi, disease in one area of the body is the product of mucus accumulation. Mucus accumulation, for example, is pneumonia, while diabetes is excess mucus in the pancreas. He argues that in an alkaline environment, diseases do not exist and begin to arise when the body is more acidic. He claims to restore the normal alkaline condition of the body and detoxify the infected body by carefully observing his routine using his expensive supplements. Originally, Dr. Sebi thought this diet could cure diseases such as HIV, sickle cell anemia, leukemia and lupus. Sebi's diet contains a trimmed-down list of items that have been endorsed by Sebi. The diet is considered a "vegan diet," the reason being that animal products are not allowed. Dr. Sebi believed that in order for the human body to heal itself, one should faithfully follow the diet for the rest of one's life. Finally, while many individuals believe that the program has healed them, no scientific findings support these claims. but still the Sebi diet plans are famous worldwide with many positive reviews available on the internet.

Because of its strong focus on a plant-based diet, this is an advantage of the Sebi diet. The diet encourages the consumption of a huge proportion of fruits and vegetables rich in fiber, vitamins, minerals and plant sources.

Significantly lower inflammation and cell proliferation, as well as defenses against many health disorders, have been linked with diets rich in fruits and vegetables. Those who consume seven or more servings of fruits and vegetables each day have a 25% to 31% lower risk of heart disease and cancer (based on a study of 65,226 individuals).

In addition, most people do not consume enough dairy products. In a 2017 survey, 9.3 percent and 12.2 percent of individuals met the fruit and vegetable guidelines, respectively. In addition, Dr. Sebi's diet encourages consumption of whole foods rich in fiber and good fats, such as nuts, beans and vegetable oils. A lower risk of heart disease has been associated with these foods.

Finally, with the overall improvement of the eating plan, health can be improved by avoiding and limiting ultra-processed foods.

Disadvantages:

This diet is extremely lacking in protein: no animal products, eggs, dairy, even soy are allowed by Sebi. She also limits many other beans and legumes. Some hemp seeds, nuts, natural growing grains, and Brazil nuts are the only things that have any protein in the diet. It can be quite difficult to meet dietary needs with just these items. Protein is a key element of every cell in the human body, and even to help create and heal tissues, the body needs protein. Muscles, skin, blood and tissues are all an important building block of protein. Nutritional deficiencies and malnutrition can result from limiting major foods and nutritional content. While it supports some fruits and vegetables, it curiously limits quite a few foods. It allows cherry and plum tomatoes, for example, but no other types. Iceberg lettuce and shiitake mushrooms are other types of food he restricts, which makes this diet much stricter, making it extremely difficult to stick to.

Sebi's main focus is on his products that make big promises of "speeding up the recovery process" and "rejuvenating and engaging intercellular development." Some packages cost well over $1,500 and don't list any nutrient specifications or quantities. This makes it difficult to understand what you'll be getting from his proprietary blends and also what exactly his supplements contain.

Above all, Dr. Sebi is not a doctor, so there is no evidence-based study to support his claims and guidelines. his extremely strict dietary recommendations promote the re-removal of major food groups that can have detrimental effects on health or, not to be forgotten, can lead to a bad relationship with food. It is important not to fall into the trap of the diet conspiracy to know the truth and make sure that every diet you adopt is vali-dated by science.

In 1993, after claiming that his diet can cure delicate situations, such as HIV, lupus and leukemia, Dr. Sebi faced a liti-gation. According to Health line, a court asked him to withdraw from making such claims. It is critical to know that there was no PhD obtained by Dr. Sebi. There was also no scientific support for his diet and nutrients. Finally, other unhealthy habits, such as consuming supplements to achieve satiety, are promoted by this diet. Since nutrients are not a significant source of energy, unhealthy eating habits are further driven by this argument.

The lack of protein and other key minerals, which are an excellent source of nutrition, are not allowed by Sebi's nutritional guide. Only nuts, some Brazil nuts, sesame seeds and hemp seeds that are not rich sources of protein are allowed. For example, 4 grams and 9 grams of protein are given by 1/4 cup (25 grams) of nuts and 3 tablespoons (30 grams) of hemp seeds, accordingly.

You'll need to eat incredibly large amounts of these foods to meet your protein intake needs.

While some foods, including potassium, beta carotene, and vitamin C and Vita-min-E, appear high in the diet, they are relatively low in omega3, iron, calcium, and vitamins D and B12, the common nutrients of concern to those on a strictly plant-based diet. Dr. Sebi's website mentions that in his products, some ingredients are patented and unspecified.

This is important, as it is not clear what nutrition you are getting and how much you are getting, it is difficult to know if you are meeting your daily nutrient requirements. Another significant problem with Dr. Sebi's diet policy is the lack of objective evi-dence to support it, not based on actual research. He states that acid development in the body is regulated by the foods and supplements mentioned in his diet.

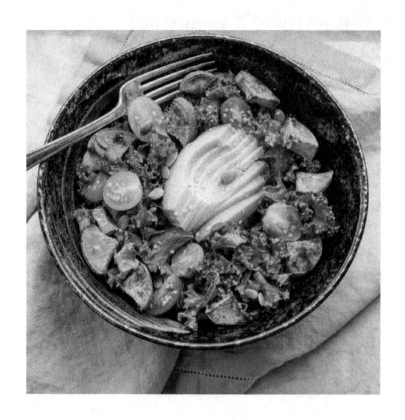

Breakfast

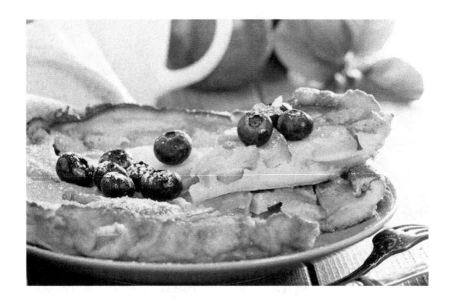

Oats Breakfast

Cooking Time: 3 minutes + refrigerating

Servings: 1

Ingredients

- 1 cup oats

- ½ cup almond milk

- 1 tablespoon cinnamon

- ½ tablespoon Pumpkin seed butter

Instructions

1. To an airtight glass jar add the oats.

2. Add milk, cinnamon and pumpkin seed butter. Mix well and close tightly.

3. Place the jar in a fridge for about 8 hours.

4. Remove from oven and pour in the serving bowl. Enjoy!

Breakfast Quinoa Porridge

Cooking Time: 10 minutes Servings: 1

Ingredients

- 1 cup quinoa, rinsed

- 2 cups water

- 1 cup coconut milk

- ¼ cup sesame and pumpkin seeds

- ½ tablespoon cinnamon

- 1 tablespoon fresh lemon zest

- Salt

Instructions

1. To a small pot add water, quinoa and salt to taste.

2. Place pot over medium heat and bring mixture to a boil.

3. Mix the coconut milk with cinnamon.

4. Pour milk mixture over the cooked quinoa, mix well until creamy. Serve porridge in bowls and top with lemon zest.

5. Enjoy topped with seeds!

Super Seed Spelt Pancakes

Cooking Time: 10 minutes

Servings: 3

Ingredients

- ¼ cup pumpkin seeds, grounded

- ¼ cup sesame seeds, grounded

- ¼ cup flax seeds, grounded

- ½ cup chia seeds, grounded

- 1 cup buckwheat groats, grounded

- 1 ½ teaspoons ground cinnamon

- ½ teaspoon baking powder

- 1 teaspoon baking soda

- ½ teaspoon stevia extract

- 2 tables almond milk

- 1 teaspoon olive oil

Instructions

1.   In a large bowl combine the pumpkin seed flour, sesame seeds flour, flax seeds flour, chia seeds flour and buckwheat groats flour.

2. Add baking powder and baking soda to flour. Mix well. Add stevia extract and almond milk.

3. Mix well to form a smooth batter.

4. Place a pan over medium heat. Add coconut oil to the pan to grease it.

5. Pour thin layers of the batter into the hot pan.

6. Cook for 3 minutes, when bubbles appear on top, flip the pancake and continue to cook the other side.

7. Serve pancakes and enjoy!

Blueberry Porridge

Cooking Time: 8 hours 30 minutes

Servings: 1

Ingredients

- ¼ cup buckwheat groats, soaked overnight

- ½ cup + 2 tablespoons pure water

- ¼ cup blueberries

- 1 tablespoon chia seeds

- 10 almonds

- ½ cups unsweetened almond milk

- ¼ teaspoon ground cinnamon

- ¼ teaspoon vanilla extract

- 1 pinch stevia

Instructions

1. To a medium bowl add the buckwheat groats.

2. Add water to the buckwheat, stir and set aside to soak for 8 hours.

3. To another bowl, add chia seeds and 2 tablespoons water for ½ an hour.

4.   Drain excess water and set aside the buckwheat, almonds and chia seeds.

5.   Place a skillet over medium high heat. Add soaked buckwheat and almond milk. Cook for minutes until creamy.

6.   To the skillet add the almonds, chia seeds, cinnamon, vanilla extract and stevia. Stir to mix well.

7.   Remove from heat and serve in serving bowls. Top with blueberries. Enjoy!

Lunch

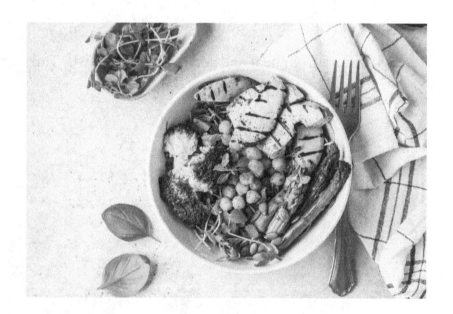

Dr. Sebi's" cleansing green soup

Serving: 4

Total Time: 1 hour

Ingredients:

• 3 if medium otherwise 2 large onions (yellow color), peeled and chopped them roughly.

• Zucchini 1, washed not peeled, and chopped roughly.

• Dandelion greens 1 bunch.

• Wild arugula1 bunch

• Vegetable broth homemade 4 cups (make it with approved vegetables only)

• Packed basil1/2 cup

• Packed dill1/2 cup

• key lime Juice of 1

• grapeseed oil 3 tbs

• sea salt 1/4 tbs

• avocado1/4

• Cayenne pepper, as per your taste

Directions:

To make this cleaning soup, begin to heat the grapeseed oil in a wide pot on medium-high heat. Add the onion and then cook for 5 mins, stirring regularly, until translucent.

Add the dandelion greens, the zucchini and the wild arugula and simmer for another 5 minutes. Put in vegetable stock (homemade) and wait for a boil, decrease heat and let it cook, cover, for 15-20 minutes. Let it cool, with lid off, for 15 minutes.

If required, combine batches of basil, dill, avocado, lime, sea salt, juice and cayenne pepper, till very smooth. Serve and change the seasonings. Decorate with some new herbs.

If you prepare Dr. Sebi's Cleansing Green Soup, you are requested to please take a photo and share with the world on Sebi 's Official page of Facebook. We love if you share your experience with us.

Bell Pepper and Roasted Tomato Soup

Serving: 2

Total Time: 50 Minutes

Ingredients:

- Ripe Roma tomatoes 4

- red bell peppers 3

- fresh sprigs thyme 3

- Vegetable broth homemade 1/4 cup (make it with approved vegetables only)

- sea salt 100% pure according to your taste and some sesame oil

Directions:

Preheat your oven at 375 degrees F. Chop the peppers in quarter then cut the cores. Slice the tomatoes and put the bell peppers onto rimmed baking dish. Drizzle completely with the sesame oil and dust with sea salt. Spread the thyme all over the vegetables. Roast for about 35-40 minutes in a heated oven. Move everything into a blender or a food pro-cessor.

Include the heated broth and the puree till it looks smooth, add more broth if required to obtain the perfect consistency. Apply salt as per your taste. Pour in the bowls and serve.

Cherry Tomato Salad

Serving: 5

Total time: 10 mins.

Ingredients:

- Cherry tomatoes 4 cups

- Red onion 1/4 cup, sliced

- Herbs like dill, sweet basil,

- Olive oil, 1/4 cup

- The Key lime juice 1 1/2 tbsp.

- Date sugar 1/4 teaspoon

- Salt as per taste

- Cayenne pepper as required

Directions:

Preparing the cherry tomato salad begins with putting the tomatoes into a wide bowl and then adding the red onion and the herbs. Now, let's bring on the dressing! Take a tiny cup, mix together the olive oil, along with the date syrup, the lime juice, the sea salt and the cayenne pepper accord-ing to taste. Add the dressing into the mixture of tomatoes and swirl gently to cover uniformly. Serve, and have fun! Have you liked this recipe? Follow Dr. Sebi's recipes and find out more ideas and information about cooking!

Headache Averting Salad

Serving: 3

Total time: 7 mins.

Ingredients:

- Seeded cucumber 1/2

- Watercress 2 cups

- Olive oil 2 tbsp.

- Key lime juice 1 tbsp.

- Cayenne pepper as per taste

- Sea salt as per taste

Directions:

Mix well the olive oil with the key lime. Arrange the watercress and the cucumber. Add the seasoning and, for taste,
spray with the salt and the pepper. Enjoy the delicious sal-ad.

Cucumber Salad (Asian Style)

Serving: 1

Total time: 5 mins.

Ingredients:

- Key lime juice three tbs.

- Sesame oil 1 tbs.

- Date sugar 1/2 tsp.

- Sea salt 1/4 tsp.

- Ginger 1 tbs., in grated form

- Sesame seeds 1 tbs.

- Seaweed 1 tbs., in powdered granulated form

Direction:

To cook the Asian Cucumber Salad, simply pour it all to-gether and enjoy it!

Avocado Basil Pasta Salad

Serving: 6

Total time: 15 mins.

Ingredients:

• Avocado 1, sliced

• Fresh basil 1 cup, sliced

• Cherry tomatoes 1-pint, cut into two halves

• Key lime juice 1 tbsp.

• Agave syrup 1 tsp.

• Olive oil 1/4 cup

• Spelt-pasta 4 cups, cooked or any other pasta, ac-cepted by Dr. Sebi's book "Cell-Food Nutritional Guide."

Directions:

In a wide tub, put the cooked pasta. Add the tomatoes, basil and avocado and stir until the components have been completely combined. In a tiny cup, blend well together with the oil, the agave syrup, the lime juice, and the sea salt. Mix with the pasta and blend to combine.

Strawberry Salad with Dandelion

Serving: 4 Total time: 50 mins.

Ingredients:

- Grape-seed oil 2 tbsp.

- Strawberries 10, must be ripe one, chopped

- Red onion one medium, chopped

- Dandelion greens 4 cups

- Key lime juice 2 tbsp.

- Sea salt as per taste

Directions:

Take a nonstick pan (of 12-inch), put grapeseed oil in it and heat it over medium flame. Now add sea salt (1 pinch) and the sliced onions in the pan. Cook, stirring regularly until the onions are smooth, softly golden and decreased to about one-third of the raw amount.In a little cup, add one tea-spoon of the key lime juice in the strawberry slices. Clean the dandelion greens and break them into bite-sized bits if you prefer. Once the onions are almost done, pour the rest of the key lime juice into the pan, then cook for a few minutes till the onions are browned. Remove the ointment from heat. In the salad cup, mix the onions, greens and strawberries along with all of the juices. Sprinkle the sea salt and enjoy.

Electric Pasta Salad (Alkaline)

Serving: 5-7

Total Time: 30 mins.

Ingredients

- Spelt Pasta/Basic Homemade Pasta 4 cups, cooked

- Bell Peppers 1 cup, either Red, Yellow or Green, cubed

- Zucchini/Summer Squash 1 cup, chopped

- Onions 1/2 cup, chopped

- Cherry Tomatoes 1/2 cup, cut them in two halves

- Black Olives 1/4 cup

- Alkaline "Garlic" Sauce 3/4 to 1 cup

Directions

Toss all the ingredients in a wide bowl once well combined and enjoy the Electric Pasta Salad (alkaline).

Chickpea Soup

Serving: 4

Total Time: 30 minutes

Ingredients:

- Chickpeas 2 cups

- Zucchini 1 small size

- Bell pepper1

- Small onion1

- Water as required

- Seasoning with own choice

Directions:

Place all things in a pot and simmer over medium heat till vegetables are aldente. As soon as the soup gets ready and vegetables are cooked, take a multi-purpose blender and then blend them well. That's the best way to enjoy that. This is going to produce a soup for a couple of days.

Orange-Spiced Pumpkin Hummus

Cooking time: 1-3 hours

Servings: 2 cups

Ingredients

- 1 tablespoon maple syrup

- cinnamon, to taste

- 3/4 cup pumpkin puree, unsweetened

- 1/4 teaspoon orange zest

- ginger, to taste

- 1 cup raw cashews, soaked overnight

- 1/4 cup warm vanilla almond milk

- nutmeg, to taste

- 1 tablespoon organic extra-virgin coconut oil, softened

Instructions

1.   Drain cashews and blend all ingredients in a blender, until smooth.

2.   Pour batter into a greased oven-friendly dish and bake for 1-3 hours or until your desired doneness, at 275 F. Serve.

Lentil Soup

Cooking time: 30 minutes Servings: 4

Ingredients

- 1/4 teaspoon sea salt, divided

- ¼ teaspoon black pepper, divide

- 2 cups sturdy greens, chopped (such as collard greens or kale)

- 2 tablespoons water

- 1 cup uncooked green or brown lentils, rinsed and drained

- 2 cloves garlic, minced

- 2-3 sprigs fresh rosemary or thyme

- 2 small shallots or 1/2 white onion, diced

- 4 cups vegetable broth plus more, if needed

- 4 large carrots, thinly sliced

- 3 cups yellow or red baby potatoes, chopped into bite-size pieces

- 4 stalks celery, thinly sliced

Optional:

- brown rice, cauliflower rice or white rice

- spelt dinner rolls

- fresh parsley

- garlic and herb flatbread

Instructions

1. Add water or oil to a preheated pot along with celery, carrots, shallots/onion, and garlic. Season with pepper and salt and stir well.

2. Sauté until veggies are golden brown and slightly tender, for 4-5 minutes. Reduce heat if garlic starts burning.

3. Add in potatoes and season again with a bit of pepper and salt. Stir and continue cooking for another 2 minutes.

4. Add rosemary or thyme and vegetable broth. Raise the heat and bring to a rolling simmer.

5. Stir in lentil, cook a bit until heated through, then turn down the heat. Simmer until potatoes and lentils are tender, for 15-20 minutes.

6. Stir in greens and cook until wilted for a few minutes, covered. Adjust the taste and add more pepper, salt and herbs, if desired.

7. If soup is too much thick, add vegetable broth.

8.   Serve delicious lentil soup as is or with the favorite servings.

9.   Garnish with parsley.

10.   Leftovers can be refrigerated for up to 5 days or store for up to a month in the freezer.

Romaine Lettuce Salad (Grilled)

Serving: 1

Total time: 30 mins.

Ingredients:

- Romaine lettuce 4 small heads, washed

- Key lime juice 1 tbsp.

- Red onion 1 tbsp., cut into fine pieces

- Onion powder as per taste

- Sea salt as per taste

- Fresh basil 1 tbsp., cut into fine pieces

- Cayenne pepper as per taste

- Agave syrup 1 tbsp.

- Olive oil 4 tbsp.

Directions:

Place the cut side of the lettuce half in a wide nonstick tray. Don't apply some oil to it. Turn over the lettuce to check its hue. Made sure that the lettuce is golden brown on both ends. Turn off the heat, remove the pan, and let the lettuce cool down on a large plate. In a tiny mixing cup, add the red onion with the olive oil, the key lime juice, the agave syrup and the new basil. Now as per taste, add the salt and pep-per. Whisk to mix it well. Take a serving dish, put the grilled lettuce into this dish. Now drizzle it with the dressing and enjoy it.

Did you like this dish? Next, try our Watercress Citrus Salad and the Alkaline-Electric Salad. Let's see which one will be your favorite.

Basic Electric Chickpea or Bengal Gram Salad ("Tuna" Salad)

Serving: 2-4 Total Time: 1 hour 15 mins.

Ingredients

- Chickpeas 2 cups, properly cooked

- Basic Electric Hemp Seed Mayo 2/3 cup

- Red Onions 1/4 cup, chopped

- Green Peppers 1/8 cup, cubed

- Dulse Granules 1 tbsp. or Nori Sheet 1/2

- Onion Powder 2 tsp.

- Dill 1 tsp.

- Sea Salt 1/4 tsp.

- Masher

Dimensions:

Take chickpeas and add into the bowl and grind until the optimal texture has been achieved. If a sheet of Nori is used, split into tiny pieces and mix with the chickpeas. Mix the remaining ingredients to the bowl and blend well. Keep it in refrigera-tor to cool for about 30 – 60 minutes before eating. Enjoy the Alkaline Electric Chickpea "Tuna" Salad!

Chunky Vegetable Soup

Cooking time: 18 minutes

Servings: 2

Ingredients

- 1 can cannellini beans

- salt and pepper, to taste

- 1 red onion, diced

- 1 ½ cups low-sodium vegetable stock

- 3 cloves garlic, diced

- 1 cup baby spinach

- 1 teaspoon dried rosemary

- 1 celery stalk, diced

- 1 teaspoon dried thyme

- 1 cup eggplant, cubed

- 4 tomatoes, roughly chopped

- 1 large zucchini, cubed

Instructions

1. Sauté celery, garlic and onion with a splash of stock until onion is translucent.

2.   Add in the remaining stock and tomatoes and simmer for a few minutes at low.

3.   Add in a cup of cubed eggplant, 1 teaspoon dried thyme, 1 teaspoon dried rosemary, and zucchini. Simmer until veggies are tender, covered.

4.   Add in a can of cannellini beans and continue simmering for another 5 minutes.

5.   Stir in spinach just before turning off the flame.

6.   Adjust pepper and salt, if desired.

Cinnamon Maple Sweet Potato Bites

Cooking time: 25 minutes

Servings: 3-4

Ingredients

- ½ teaspoon cornstarch

- 1 teaspoon cinnamon

- 4 medium sweet potatoes, peeled and cut into bite-size cubes

- 2-3 tablespoons maple syrup

- 3 tablespoons butter, melted

Instructions

1. Line the baking sheet with parchment paper.

2. Add potatoes cubes to a gallon-sized bag and add in 3 tablespoons melted butter. Shake well until all pieces are coated with butter.

3. Add in 2-3 tablespoons maple syrup, 1 teaspoon cinnamon, and ½ teaspoon cornstarch. Shake the bag again until all pieces are coated, then transfer to a prepared baking

sheet, making sure that they do not stack over each other. Do in batches, if desired.

4.   Sprinkle cinnamon over top, if desired and bake in a preheated oven at 425 F, for about 25-30 minutes, stirring about halfway through in the cooking time.

5.   Once done, take them out and allow to cool.

6.   Serve.

Cauliflower Soup

Cooking time: 35 minutes

Servings: 3 to 4

Ingredients

- 1 13 oz. can of filtered water

- fresh dill

- 2 tablespoons olive oil

- fresh cracked pepper

- 1 1/2 cups sweet white onion, finely chopped

- dash of olive oil

- 2 large cloves of garlic, finely chopped

- 1 tablespoon arrowroot powder

- 1 head of cauliflower, cut into florets

- 2 tablespoons nutritional yeast

- season, to taste

- 1 teaspoon vegetable stock paste

- 1 13 oz. can of coconut milk

Instructions

1. Preheat olive oil in a large pot for 20 seconds.

2.   Add onion and sauté for about 10 minutes, until translucent and caramelized, stirring often.

3.   Add garlic and continue sautéing for another 5 minutes.

4.   Add cauliflower florets, season to taste and cook for 5-7 minutes, stirring often.

5.   Raise the heat and add water, coconut milk, nutritional yeast, and stock paste.

6.   Put on the lid and bring to a boil. Once boiled, turn down the heat and simmer until cauliflower is softened.

7.   Add ¼ cup water to a small bowl along with 1 tablespoon arrowroot powder. Stir well, then add to the soup mixture slowly and gradually.

8.   Blend the soup mixture in a high speed blender for a minute.

9.   Transfer to a serving bowl and serve with dill, dash of lemon, cracked pepper and olive oil.

White Bean Cauliflower Curry Soup

Cooking time: 25 minutes

Servings: 4

Ingredients

- 1/2 (14-oz.) can navy beans, drained and rinsed

- 1/2 teaspoon chili powder

- 1/2 white onion, finely chopped

- 1/4 teaspoon ground coriander

- 4 garlic cloves, minced

- 1/2 tablespoon curry powder

- 2 tablespoons fresh ginger, peeled and minced

- 2 cups low-sodium vegetable stock

- 1/2 head cauliflower, coarsely chopped

- 1/2 (14-oz) can coconut milk

Instructions

1. Add all ingredients to a stockpot and bring to a boil.

Turn the heat down and simmer until cauliflower is softened,

for around 25 minutes.

2.   Puree soup in an immersion blender until smooth. Serve.

Dinner

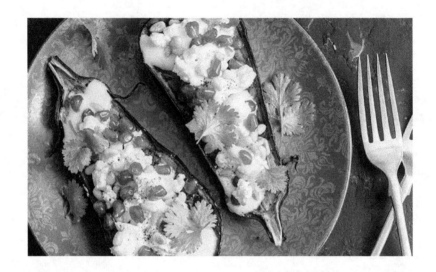

Pantry Dal

Cook Time: 25 minutes

Servings: 4

Ingredients:

- 4 cups veggies, peeled and diced
- 1 heaping tablespoon olive oil
- ½ cup water
- ½ cup red lentils, uncooked
- 14 oz. light coconut milk
- 14 oz. diced tomatoes
- 1 ½ teaspoons minced onion
- 1 ½ teaspoons garlic powder
- 1 tablespoon curry powder
- 1 teaspoon fine sea salt
- black pepper
- rice, cooked

Instructions:

1. Melt coconut oil over low medium heat in a pot. Peel and dice veggies into ½" pieces. Add to pot and stir well then increase heat to medium.

2.　　Add diced tomatoes with juices, water, lentils, all the spices, coconut milk, salt and pepper and stir until well combined.

3.　　Increase the heat to high and bring to a low boil. Reduce the heat to medium and cook for 30 minutes, uncovered. Stir frequently.

4.　　Serve with rice.

Cherry Crisp

Cooking time: 45 minutes Servings: 10

Ingredients

For the filling:

- 2 tablespoons + 1 teaspoon arrowroot starch or tapioca

- 1 tablespoon lemon juice

- 1 1/2 lbs. cherries, pitted and halved

- 1 teaspoon pure vanilla extract

- 1/4 cup maple sugar or coconut sugar

For the topping:

- 1/2 cup unsweetened coconut, shredded

- 1/4 teaspoon sea salt

- 1/4 cup maple sugar or coconut sugar

- 1 teaspoon cinnamon

- 1 cup blanched almond flour

- 1 teaspoon pure vanilla extract

- 2/3 cup raw almonds

- 1/4 cup + 2 tablespoons coconut oil soft but solid

Instructions

To prepare the topping:

1.   Add 2/3 cup raw almonds to a processor and pulse until you have lager crumbs.

2.   Add in 1/4 cup maple sugar or coconut sugar, 1 cup blanched almond flour, 1 teaspoon pure vanilla extract, 1/2 cup shredded coconut, 1/4 teaspoon sea salt, and 1/4 teaspoon sea salt.

3.   Pulse or stir in coconut oil until slightly pasty/crumbly but avoid overmixing.

4.   Place in a refrigerator.

To prepare the filling:

1.   Add all the filing ingredients to a bowl and stir well until combined and transfer to a pie or baking dish.

2.   Crumble the topping over the cherries and bake in a preheated oven at 350 F, until topping is golden brown, for about 40-45 minutes.

3.   Top with coconut vanilla ice cream and serve.

Wild Rice Tabbouleh

Cook Time: 1 hour Servings: 4

Ingredients:

- 8 cups cold water

- 1 cup wild rice

- 2 cups seeded cucumber, diced and peeled

- 2 cups tomatoes, diced

- 2 tablespoons olive oil

- 2 tablespoons lemon juice

- ¼ cup parsley, chopped

- ¼ cup mint, chopped

- sea salt

Instructions:

1. Cover rice with water in a large pan. Add 1 teaspoon salt and bring to boil. Cover and cook for 1 hour over moderately low heat. Drain rice well.

2. Toss rice with cucumber, tomatoes, oil, mint, lemon juice and parsley. Season with salt.Serve.

Cucumber Dill Dressing

Serving: 2

Total time: 3 mins.

Ingredients:

- Chopped Plum Tomatoes, 2

- Sesame Seeds2 tbsp.

- Minced Onion, 1 tbsp.

- Agave 1 tbsp.

- Lime Juice 1 tbsp.

- Minced Ginger, 1 tsp.

Directions:

Start by blending all the ingredients in a blender and blend them for about 1&half minute, it is now ready to serve.

Chili Garlic Tofu with Sesame Broccolini

Cook Time: 15 minutes

Servings: 2

Ingredients:

- 12 oz. extra firm tofu
- ½ teaspoon pepper corms, fresh cracked
- 2 tablespoons peanut oil
- 4 garlic cloves, smashed
- ½ teaspoon salt
- 8 oz. broccolini
- 2 tablespoons honey
- 1 tablespoon chili garlic sauce
- 1 ½ teaspoons soy sauce
- 1 tablespoon sesame seeds, toasted
- 2 small sheets roasted seaweed, sliced into thin strips

Instructions:

1. Drain and blot tofu and cut into ½" thick pieces. Blot again.

2. Heat oil in a skillet over medium heat. Add smashed garlic, salt and pepper and swirl and cook for 2 minutes.

3. Cook tofu in the same skillet over medium heat for 5 minutes each side.

4. Fill a medium pot with ¾" water and set on stove. Place a steam basket inside and layer it with broccolini. Cover and bring to boil. Steam for 5 minutes.

5. Mix honey, chili sauce and soy sauce in a bowl and set aside. Cut seaweed strips.

6. Divide tofu among 2 plates and take the garlic out of the skillet, transfer broccolini to the skillet and stir to coat well.

7. Add toasted sesame seeds and cook for 1 minute over medium heat. Divide among the plates.

8. Add chili sauce to the tofu and top with seaweed strands.

9. Serve.

Thai Red Tofu and Sweet Potato Curry

Cook Time: 25 minutes

Servings: 4

Ingredients:

- 9/10 lb. firm tofu

- 2 cups boiling water

- 1 cup jasmine rice

- 1 tablespoon olive oil

- 7/10 lb. sweet potato, peeled and cut into 1/2 inch

- 1 red bell pepper, diced

- 3 tablespoons red Thai curry paste

- ¾ cup baby sweetcorn, sliced

- 1 lime juice

- 2 cups coconut milk

- ¾ cup mangetout peas

- 2 tablespoons coriander leaves

- salt

Instructions:

1.	Press the tofu firmly, drain for 10 minutes and chop into bite-sized pieces.

2.	Add jasmine rice to a pan and add the boiling water and a pinch salt. Cover and bring to boil, turn down the heat to low and cook for 8 minutes. Take rice off the heat but leave the lid on. Let it rest for 5 minutes.

3.	Heat 1 tablespoon oil in a pan, add tofu and stir fry for 3 minutes.

4.	Add red pepper, sweet potato and sweet corn and fry for 1 minute.

5.	Add red curry paste and fry for 1 more minute.

6.	Add 1 cup coconut milk and bring to boil. Cover with a lid and cook for 8 minutes. Add more coconut milk if required.

7.	Add the meangetout peas, lime juice and a pinch salt and cook for 1 minute.

8.	Add coriander on top and serve curry with cooked rice.

Vegetable Omelet

Serving: 1

Total Time: 25 minutes

Ingredients:

- Oregano ¼ tsp.

- Flour (Garbanzo Beans) ¼ cup

- Chopped Mushrooms ¼ cup

- Chopped Roma Tomato, ¼ cup

- Diced Green Pepper, ¼ cup

- Chopped Onion ¼ cup,

- Sea Salt 100% Pure ¼ tsp.

- Grapeseed Oil 1 tbsp.

- Onion Powder ¼ tsp

- Spring Water 1/3 cup

- Basil, sweet ¼ tsp.

- Cayenne Powder ¼ tsp.

Directions:

Start by putting garbanzo bean flour, include water and add seasoning in a wide mixing bowl. Whisk the combination properly, so it is properly blended. Heat oil in a large skillet on medium-high heat. When the oil is warmed, mix in a spoonful of all vegetables and the tomatoes. Sautee it for 2-3 minutes or before it becomes slightly tender.

Now add the flour mixture over it and blend it properly. Cook the mixture for 4 minutes, then turn mixture side by side. Using a spatula, remove the omelet's sides and turn it gently to the elevated position such that all parts of the omelet can be lifted. Only get fried. Serve them warm, please.

Energy Balls

Serving: 1

Total Time: 20 minutes

Ingredients:

- Salt ¼ tsp.

- Brazil Nuts ¾ cup; Coconut Oil 2 tbsp.

- Walnuts ¾ cup; Dried Fruits ¼ cup

- Sesame Seeds ½ cup; Hemp Hearts ½ cup, Figs ½ cup, dried

Directions:

Start by putting the seeds (sesame), figs, salt in the food processor and Mix them all for 2-3 minutes or till a sticky blend is produced. Shift to a tub.

Put Brazil nuts and walnuts in the processor and then mix till they convert into a texture yet crumbly. Add the walnut blend to the mixture with sesame seeds.

Merge and mix with spoon in the fruits or hemp hearts until mixed. Mix and Combine the mixture with coconut. Finally, create rolls from the blend and store them all in air-tight jar.

Macaroni & Cheese

Serving: 10

Total Time: 45 minutes

Ingredients:

- Grapeseed Oil 2 tsp.

- Alkaline Pasta 12 oz.

- Juice 1 of ½ Key Lime

- Onion Powder 2 tsp.

- Garbanzo Flour ¼ cup

- Sea Salt 1 tsp.

- Spring Water 1 cup

- Raw Brazil Nuts 1 cup, overnight soaked

- Hempseed Milk 1 cup

- Achiote, grounded ½ tsp.

Directions:

Cook the pasta first according to the directions on the pack-et. Then, heat the oven to 350 F. Place the cooked pasta and drizzle oil over it into a baking dish. In a high-speed mixer, put all remaining ingredients and mix until the sauce gets creamy for 2 min or until ticked. Stir the cooked pasta with the sauce and chop it properly. Bake pasta for 20-30 minutes.

Baked Kale Chips

Serving: 4

Total Time: 20 minutes.

Ingredients:

*	Kale 1 lb, washed & patted dry

*	Sea Salt Pure, as needed

*	Grapeseed Oil, 1 tbsp.

*	as needed, Cayenne Pepper

Directions:

Preheat your oven to 350 degrees F. Tear off leaves from kale and stem; after that place grapeseed oil, kale leaves, cayenne pepper and sea salt in the mixture. Add everything to a mixing bowl. Soak the kale leaves with seasoning and then put them for baking on the Parchment-paper-lined sheet. Next, cook for eight minutes or till they get crispy.

Macaroni & Cheese

Serving: 8-10

Total Time: 15 minutes

Ingredients:

- Hemp Milk, 1 cup

- Kamut Pasta, 12 oz.

- Pure Sea Salt, 1 tsp.

- All Spice, ½ tsp.

- Flour of Garbanzo Bean, ¼ cup.

- Brazil Nuts ½ lb, raw & soaked

- ½ Juice of 1 Lime

- Spring Water, 1 cup

- Onion Powder, 2 tsp.

- Grape-seed Oil, 2 tsp.

Directions:

Cook the pasta to render this balanced food by following Instructions as given on the packet. Preheat your oven to 350 ° F. Then, using a high-speed blender, put all the ingredi-ents required to produce the dressing. Blend the mixture for 2 minutes or before it becomes all smooth. Now, over medi-umhigh flame, heat oil in a broad skillet. Mix the pasta and simmer for 1 minute until the oil becomes hot.

Next, add the sauce over the skillet and give it all a gentle swirl. Lastly, cook pasta for about 30 minutes or till it's fully cooked.

Alkaline Electric Zucchini Bacon

Serving: 2-4

Total Time: 2 hours

Ingredients:

- Zucchini 2-3

- Date Sugar 1/4 cup

- Spring Water 1/4 cup

- Agave 2 tbsp.

- Sea Salt Smoked 1 tbsp.

- Onion Powder 1 tbsp.

- Liquid Smoke 1 tsp.

- Cayenne Powder 1/2 tsp.

- Ginger Powder 1/2 tsp.

- Mandoline / Potato Peeler

- Paper Parchment

- Grapeseed Oil

Directions:

Add all the ingredients into the saucepan and steam over low heat, and wait till they dissolved. Chop the zucchini and use the potato peeler to create the strips. In a wide bowl, mix the zucchini with the saucepan's ingredients and mari-nate for 30 to 60 minutes. There is no need for more water since it will come from zucchini. Use parchment paper on to the baking sheet and cover slightly with grape-seed oil. Cov-er the sheet with marinated strips, and bake at 400 ° F for ten minutes. Flip zucchini strips, cook 3-4 minutes, then leave to cool. If you like any of the strips to be crispy, roast for few more minutes or fry in a finely oiled pan for 30 sec. Enjoy the Alkaline-Electric-Bacon of Zucchini.

Mango Papaya Seed Dressing

Serving: 2

Total time: 3 mins.

- Ingredients
- Chopped Mango, 1 cup
- Grapeseed Oil 1/4 cup
- Lime Juice 2 tbsp.
- Ground Papaya Seed 1 tsp.
- Agave 1 tsp.
- Basil 1 tsp.
- Onion Powder 1 tsp.
- Sea Salt 1/4 tsp.

Directions:

Blend the ingredients inside blender and blend them for about a minute, it is now ready to serve.

Souces

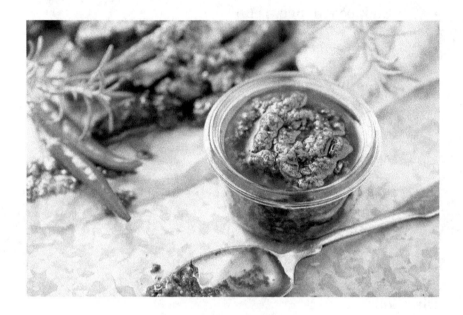

Zucchini Bread

Serving: 2

Total Time: 45 minutes

Ingredients:

- Oil 2 tbsp.

- Zucchini Puree 1 cup

- Spelt Flour 1 cup

- Pinch of Salt

- Perrier 1 tbsp.

Directions:

Start mixing the puree with the rice, milk, salt and the Per-rier spelt. Until all comes together into a large mixing bowl, pour some more water to obtain a dense and smooth dough. Now stretched the dough on a grated paper baker sheet. Bake the dough at 350 F for 33 mins. Or until cooked.

Spelt Bread

Serving: 4 Total Time: 1 hour & 10 minutes

Ingredients:

- Pure Sea Salt 2 tsp.

- Spelt Flour 4 ½ cup

- Agave Syrup ¼ cup

- Sesame Seeds 1 tsp.

- Grape Seed Oil 2 tsp.

- Spring Water 2 cups

Directions:

First, put the spelt-flour with sea salt into a food processor for 10-20 seconds. Add agave syrup and blend properly. Then add a spoon of oil and some water to get dough, then steadily mix. Process this dough for another five minutes. Holding the dough in the aggregated and distorted loaf. Preheat an oven to 350 F. Allow it to stay for 1 hour. Final-ly, bake until golden brown for 50- 60 minutes.

Chickpeas Cornbread

Serving: 14

Total Time: 25 minutes

Ingredients:

- Chickpea Flour 2 cup

- Brazil Nut Milk 1 cup

- Applesauce 1 cup

- Water, as required

- Grapeseed Oil ½ cup

- Pepper 1 tbsp.

Directions:

Start combining in large mixing bowl all necessary ingredients for making the cornbread smooth. It should be moderately consistent. If the batter is too thickened, you may also use water to dilute it. Place the grapefruit oil in the pot and add the butter to it.

Disseminate it uniformly. Bake for 28-30 minutes or till toothpick comes out clean if inserted in the batter. Cut into squares until cooled. After it gets cool, slice into squares.

Mango salsa

Serving: 3

Total Time: 10 minutes

Ingredients:

- Plum Tomatoes, 6

- Cayenne Pepper ½ tsp.

- Tomatillo 1

- Sea Salt1 tsp

- chopped Red Onion ½ cup,

- Onion Powder 1 tsp

- Green Bell Pepper ¼ cup

- Cilantro ½ cup

- ½ cup Mango,

- Juice of a half Lemon

Directions:

Start by mixing all required ingredients except salsa into the food processor with pineapple. Treat them for 10-15 sec-onds; add the mango then. Scrap the sides, mix again for 20 seconds. Take a cup and enjoy.

Avocado Yoghurt Sauce

Serving: 2

Total Time: 10 minutes

Ingredients:

- Agave Syrup 1/3 cup

- Ripe Avocado 1,

- Spring Water ¾ cup

- Juice of 2 Limes

- Berries 1 cup

Directions:

Begin with agave sipping, berries, spring water, and lime juice.

Use a high-speed mixer with avocado in it. Blend it for 1-2

minutes, till no chunks or until smooth. Serve when cooled.

Alkaline Electric Breadsticks

Serving: 2

Total Time: 45 minutes

Ingredients:

- Spelt Flour 2 cups

- spring Water3/4 cup

- Alkaline "Garlic" Sauce* 1/2 cup

- Agave 2 tsp.

- Onion Powder 1 tbsp.

- Sea Salt half of 1 tsp.

- Oregano 1 tsp.

- Basil 1 tsp.

- Grounded Brazil Nuts 1/4 cup (Optional)

- Garlic sauce, 1/4 cup in 2 cups separately.

Directions:

Add the flour to the mixer and blend for 30 seconds. Put agave into the mixer, knead the pasta for 5 minutes, and then add 1/4 cup of alkaline garlic sauce with water. Wrap in plastic lightly flour dough ball, let the dough stay for 30 minutes. Remove a small portion of the dough using a dough cutter, roll it back and forth with soft hands. Put to-gether dough ends, twist until long enough, and then posi-tion it on a bakery pan. Brush the 1/4 cup of alkaline 'garlic' sauce gently on the breadsticks and bake for 15 min, at 350 ° F.

Grind with coffee grinder the Brazil nuts until it is finely ground. Once brushed, add the remaining sauce into the breadsticks, now top with ground Brazil nozzles and bake for 3 minutes. Enjoy your fresh Electric Alkaline Breadstick.

Dessert

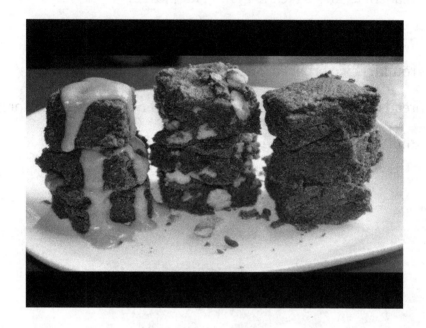

Blueberry Cake

Serving: 6

Total time: 55 mins.

Ingredients:

- Chickpea Flour 1 cup

- Blueberries 1 cup

- Spelt Flour 2/3 cup + 1 tbsp.

- Sea Salt a pinch

- Water ¾ cup

- Grapeseed Oil 2 tbsp

- Agave Nectar 6 tbsp.

Directions

First, put all the ingredients you need to cook in a blender, then blend for three minutes until there are no more chunks in it. Next, move the paste to parchment baking pan which must be proper paper-lined and distribute it uniformly. Bake for about twenty-eight to thirty minutes or when gold-en browned and baked. Enjoy!

Citrus Olive Oil Cake

Cooking time: 55 minutes Servings: 1 cake

Ingredients

For the cake:

- ¼ cup fresh citrus juice

- ½ cup extra-virgin olive oil

- 1 ½ cups regular whole wheat flour or white whole wheat flour

- ½ teaspoon pure vanilla extract

- 2 teaspoons baking powder

- 3 eggs

- ¼ teaspoon salt

- ¾ cup plain whole-milk yogurt

- 2 teaspoons citrus zest

For the glaze (optional):

- 2-3 teaspoons fresh citrus juice

- ⅓ cup powdered sugar

InstructionsButter and flour the loaf pan.Whisk together 2 teaspoons baking powder, 1 ½ cups flour, and ¼ teaspoon salt in a bowl. Rub sugar with zest in a separate bowl until sugar takes on the color. Whisk in ¾ cup yogurt, ¼ cup fresh citrus juice, ½ teaspoon pure vanilla extract, and 3 eggs until well blended. Add dry ingredients to a bowl with wet ingredients and whisk gently, until incorporated.Fold in ½ cup olive oil by using a spatula until well incorporated. Pour into a prepared pan and smooth evenly. Bake in a preheated oven at 350 F, until top is golden, for about 50-55 minutes. Tester inserted should come out clear. Once done, let it cool for 10 to 15 minutes. Run a sharp knife around edges and unmold by placing a large plate upside down over your pan and turning over carefully. Flip over and allow to cool further.Whisk together 2-3 teaspoons fresh citrus juice and ⅓ cup powdered sugar and drizzle back and forth over the cake. It may take 15 minutes to set.Slice and serve.

Blueberry Spelt Pancakes

Serving: 2

Total time: 20 mins.

Ingredients:

- Spelt Flour 2 cups

- Sea Moss ¼ tsp.

- Hemp Milk 1 cup

- Agave Syrup ½ cup

- Spring Water ½ cup

- Blueberries ½ cup

- Grapeseed Oil 2 tbsp.

Directions

For this balanced breakfast dish, add the spelled flour, the agave syrup, the sea moss and the grapeseed oil uniformly in a big mixing pot. Now, slowly pour the hemp milk into it and the water into it. Then gently press in the blueberries. After that, heat a broad pan over medium-high flame. Once the pan is hot, spray it with oil. Then, add a spoon full of the mixture and cook every side for about 3 to 5 minutes. Now finally, serve them hot.

Banana Nut Muffins

Serving: 12 slices

Total time: 50 mins.

Ingredients:

- Spelt Flour 3 ½ cup

- Bananas 3, mash them

- Spring Water, as desired

- Walnuts 1 cup, sliced

- Salt a Pinch

- Date Syrup 1 tbsp.

- Perrier ¾ cup

Directions

To produce this wonderful cake, add the mashed banana and the date syrup in the bowl and mix it until well. Mix in spelled flour, then add salt and mix until combined.

Mix it again. And mix the Perrier and the walnuts. Stir it well. If the batter appears to be too dense, add a little water as required. Now add the mixture into the molds of the muffin and line them with 3/4. Lastly, bake at 350 p.m. for about eighteen to twenty minutes or till it is bake.

Strawberry Sorbet

Servings: 4

Total Time: 4 hours 10 minutes

Ingredients:

- Date Sugar ½ cup

- Strawberries 2 cups

- Spring Water 2 cups

- Spelt Flour 1 ½ tsp.

Directions:

Begin by combing date sugar, spelled flour, and spring wa-ter in a medium-sized pot. Next, heat the mixture over low heat and cook for 8 to 10 minutes or till thickened. After that, take off the pot from the heat and allow it to cool. Once cooled, puree the strawberries in a blender. Now, mix the strawberry puree to the flour mixture and give everything a good stir. Then, pour the mixture into a container and keep it in the freezer. Cut the frozen sorbet to pieces and place it in the blender or food processor. Blend until smooth and re-turn the container to the refrigerator for a minimum of 4 hours. Finally, serve the chilled strawberry sorbet.

Strawberry Ice Cream

Servings: 3 to 4

Total Time: 6 hours 10 Minutes

Ingredients:

*   Hemp Milk ¼ cup

*   frozen strawberries, 1 cup

*   Agave Syrup 1 tbsp.

*   frozen Baby Bananas, 5

*   ripe Avocado, ½ of 1

Directions:

Place all ingredients necessary to make this ice cream into a high-speed blender. Mix them for 2-3 minutes or till the mixture is smooth. Check for sugar and, if appropriate, in-sert more agave syrup. Finally, move to the freezer-friendly jar and freeze for 4-6 hours

Lunchbox Chocolate Chip Cookies

Cooking time: 25 minutes

Servings: 24 cookies

Ingredients

- 2 teaspoons pure vanilla extract

- ½ cup grain-sweetened chocolate chips

- 1/3 cup unsweetened applesauce

- ¼ cup whole wheat pastry flour or sorghum flour

- 1/3 cup almond butter

- ½ teaspoon salt

- ½ cup dry sweetener or use vegan cane sugar/maple sugar/date sugar

- ½ teaspoon baking soda

- 1 tablespoon ground flaxseeds

- 1 1/3 cups oat flour

Instructions

1. Line two baking sheets with parchment paper.

2. Beat together ⅓ cup applesauce, ½ cup dry sweetener, ⅓ cup almond butter, and 1 tablespoon ground flaxseeds in a bowl by using a fork, until smooth.

3. Next, stir in 2 teaspoons pure vanilla extract.

4. Mix in ½ teaspoon baking soda, 1⅓ cups oat flour, and ½ teaspoon salt.

5. Add ½ cup chocolate chips and ¼ cup sorghum flour and mix well.

6. Drop spoonfuls (about 1 ½-tablespoon scoops) of this batter onto prepared sheets, about 2 inches apart. Flatten cookies to thick discs.

7. Bake in a preheated oven at 350°F, for 8-10 minutes.

8. Once done, take them out and allow to cool.

Walnut Date Nog

Servings: 2

Total Time: 10 Minutes

Ingredients:

- chopped Walnuts, ¼ cup

- Sea Salt ½ tsp.

- soaked Dates 4

- grounded Clove 1

- Hemp Seeds 4 tbsp.

- Dash of Anise

- Agave Syrup 2 tbsp.

- Spring Water 18 oz.

Directions:

Start by putting all the ingredients required to create the nog, except the clove and anise, inside a high-speed blend-er. Blend for about three minutes or till the mixture is smooth. Next, move the mixture into a medium-sized saucepan and heat. Serve with a slice of clove or anise. En-joy it.

Mango Cheesecake

Servings: 8

Total Time: 4 Hour 30 Minute

Ingredients:

- Walnut Milk 1 ½ cup

- Brazil Nuts 2 cups

- Pure Sea Salt ¼ tsp.

- Dates 6

- Lime Juice 2 tbsp.

- Sea Moss 1 tbsp.

- Agave Syrup ¼ cup

For crust:

- Agave Syrup 1/4 cup

- Sea Salt ¼ tsp.

- quartered Dates 1 ½ cup,

- Coconut Flakes 1 ½ cup

Directions:

First, put all the ingredients necessary to make the dough into a food processor, then process for 30 -45 minutes. Place the mixture onto the parchment paper-lined baking dish. Now distribute the mixture uniformly over the sheet. Then place mango slices over the crust and put it inside the freezer for 8-10 minutes. Meanwhile, put filling ingredients into a high-speed blender. Blend until the mixture is smooth. Next, dump the mixture all over the frozen surface and let it stay in the refrigerator for 3-4 hours. Finally, be-fore serving, garnish with some more slices of mango and strawberries